YUVARAJ AR
JAYAKUMAR JAYADURKA
ELAVARASI E

Aquarium fishes diagnosis and treatment with pharmaceutical drugs

YUVARAJ AR
JAYAKUMAR JAYADURKA
ELAVARASI E

Aquarium fishes diagnosis and treatment with pharmaceutical drugs

therapeutically supports and health system

LAP LAMBERT Academic Publishing

Imprint
Any brand names and product names mentioned in this book are subject to trademark, brand or patent protection and are trademarks or registered trademarks of their respective holders. The use of brand names, product names, common names, trade names, product descriptions etc. even without a particular marking in this work is in no way to be construed to mean that such names may be regarded as unrestricted in respect of trademark and brand protection legislation and could thus be used by anyone.

Cover image: www.ingimage.com

Publisher:
LAP LAMBERT Academic Publishing
is a trademark of
Dodo Books Indian Ocean Ltd. and OmniScriptum S.R.L publishing group

120 High Road, East Finchley, London, N2 9ED, United Kingdom
Str. Armeneasca 28/1, office 1, Chisinau MD-2012, Republic of Moldova, Europe
Managing Directors: Ieva Konstantinova, Victoria Ursu
info@omniscriptum.com

Printed at: see last page
ISBN: 978-620-9-37367-1

ABSTRACT:

Aquarium fish health management is a crucial component of both ornamental fish keeping and commercial aquaculture. Diseases in aquarium fishes arise primarily due to poor water quality, overcrowding, nutritional deficiencies, parasitic infestations, bacterial and fungal infections, and viral outbreaks. Early diagnosis plays a key role in minimizing mortality and preventing disease spread. Clinical signs such as abnormal swimming behavior, color changes, fin erosion, gill movement variations, and external lesions serve as important indicators for preliminary visual diagnosis. Laboratory techniques including microscopic examination of skin and gill scrapings, bacterial culture, histopathology, and advanced molecular tools like PCR and ELISA improve diagnostic accuracy and decision-making.Pharmaceutical interventions are commonly employed for targeted treatment once the causative agent is identified. Antibiotics such as oxytetracycline, erythromycin, and enrofloxacin are used for bacterial diseases like fin rot and columnaris, while antifungal drugs including malachite green, methylene blue, and potassium permanganate are effective against fungal infections. Antiparasitic agents such as formalin, praziquantel, metronidazole, and copper sulfate are widely used to control protozoans and helminths. Supportive therapy using salt baths, vitamin supplementation, and probiotics enhances recovery and strengthens immune response. However, rational drug use with correct dosage, quarantine protocols, and withdrawal periods is essential to prevent antimicrobial resistance and toxicity risks.

Keywords: Aquarium fish diseases, Diagnosis, Pharmaceutical drugs, Treatment, Water quality management.

CHAPTER 1:

INTRODUCTION TO FISH HEALTH AND AQUACULTURE

1.1 OVERVIEW OF AQUACULTURE SYSTEMS AND PRACTICES

Aquaculture, commonly referred to as fish farming, is the controlled cultivation of aquatic organisms such as fish, crustaceans, mollusks, and aquatic plants under managed environmental conditions. It represents one of the fastest-growing food production sectors in the world and plays a vital role in food security, livelihood enhancement, and economic development. As global fish demand continues to rise due to population growth, changing dietary preferences, and declining wild fish stocks, aquaculture has become a critical solution to bridge the gap between supply and demand while ensuring sustainable utilization of aquatic resources.The term *aquaculture system* encompasses the physical, biological, and management components used to raise aquatic species. These systems are designed to provide optimal conditions for growth, reproduction, and health, while maintaining water quality and minimizing environmental impact. Aquaculture practices vary widely depending on factors such as species cultured, environmental conditions, available resources, and the level of technological sophistication. Broadly, aquaculture systems can be classified into extensive, semi-intensive, and intensive systems based on the degree of control, input usage, and productivity.

Extensive aquaculture systems rely primarily on the natural productivity of the water body. Fish are stocked in ponds, lagoons, or coastal enclosures where they feed mainly on naturally available food such as plankton, algae, and detritus. Minimal human intervention is involved beyond stocking, basic monitoring, and harvesting. These systems are commonly used for low-value species and are considered environmentally friendly due to their low input requirements. However, productivity per unit area is generally low, and disease management is more difficult because of limited control over environmental parameters. Extensive systems are prevalent in rural or developing regions where resources and technology are limited but where land and water availability are abundant.

Semi-intensive aquaculture systems represent an intermediate approach, combining natural productivity with supplementary feeding and controlled management. In these systems, pond fertilization using organic or inorganic materials is employed to boost plankton growth, while formulated feeds are provided to enhance growth rates. Water exchange and aeration are occasionally used to maintain suitable water quality. Semi-intensive systems allow higher stocking densities and improved yields compared to extensive systems. They are common in commercial fish farming operations, especially for species such as tilapia, carp, and catfish. The moderate level of input also makes semi-intensive systems economically feasible while maintaining environmental sustainability if properly managed.

Intensive aquaculture systems are highly controlled environments designed for maximum productivity. Fish are stocked at very high densities and rely entirely on nutritionally complete formulated feeds. These systems utilize continuous aeration, filtration, and water quality management to support optimal growth and health. Intensive systems are technologically sophisticated and include recirculating aquaculture systems (RAS), raceways, tanks, and cages. They are capable of producing large quantities of fish in limited space, making them suitable for urban or resource-limited areas. However, they require significant capital investment, technical expertise, and energy input. Waste management and disease control are critical challenges in intensive systems due to high organic loading and close contact among fish.Among modern intensive systems, **Recirculating Aquaculture Systems (RAS)** have gained prominence due to their efficiency and sustainability potential. RAS continuously treat and reuse water within the system using mechanical and biological filtration, thereby minimizing water consumption and environmental discharge. This technology allows aquaculture to occur in areas with limited water resources and provides a high degree of control over temperature, oxygen, and waste removal. Despite the advantages, RAS operations require high initial investment, continuous power supply, and skilled management to ensure profitability.

Cage culture systems are another widely practiced intensive form of aquaculture, particularly in lakes, reservoirs, and coastal waters. Fish are confined in floating cages made of netting material, allowing free exchange of water while retaining the cultured species. Cage culture enables efficient use of existing water bodies without the need for land-based ponds and allows easy monitoring and feeding. However, it poses risks of disease transmission, environmental pollution from uneaten feed and waste, and conflicts with other water users. Sustainable cage culture requires proper site selection, feeding management, and adherence to environmental regulations.

Integrated Multi-Trophic Aquaculture (IMTA) and **polyculture systems** are gaining attention as environmentally sustainable practices. These systems involve culturing multiple species from different trophic levels in the same environment, where the waste from one species serves as input for another. For instance, fish can be cultured alongside shellfish and seaweeds, which utilize dissolved nutrients and particulate waste. This integration improves resource utilization, reduces pollution, and enhances ecological balance. Similarly, rice-fish culture and livestock-fish integrated systems have been practiced traditionally in Asia for centuries, offering both economic and environmental benefits.Aquaculture practices also differ based on **habitat type**—freshwater, brackish water, or marine. Freshwater aquaculture typically includes species such as carp, tilapia, and catfish, often cultured in ponds or tanks. Brackish water aquaculture is prominent in coastal regions, focusing on species like shrimp and milkfish. Marine aquaculture, or mariculture, involves species such as salmon, sea bass, oysters, and mussels, and is usually conducted in offshore cages or coastal enclosures. Each habitat presents unique management challenges, including water salinity, temperature fluctuations, and disease risks.Technological advances have significantly transformed aquaculture practices. The development of high-quality feeds, automated feeding systems, water quality sensors, biosecurity measures, and genetic improvement programs has enhanced efficiency and sustainability. Selective breeding and biotechnology have led to improved growth rates, disease resistance, and feed conversion efficiency in cultured species. Likewise, advances in digital monitoring, artificial intelligence, and data analytics are enabling precision aquaculture, where farmers can optimize feeding, water quality, and health management in real time.Sustainability remains a central focus in modern aquaculture. Unsustainable practices such as overuse of antibiotics, poor waste management, and habitat destruction have led to environmental concerns in the past. Consequently, there is an increasing shift toward **eco-friendly aquaculture**, incorporating biofloc technology, aquaponics, and renewable energy use. **Biofloc technology (BFT)** utilizes microbial communities to recycle nutrients and maintain water quality, reducing dependence on water exchange and feed costs. **Aquaponics**, which combines aquaculture with hydroponic plant production, represents a closed-loop system that maximizes resource efficiency and minimizes waste.Socioeconomic aspects of aquaculture are equally important. The industry provides employment opportunities for millions of people worldwide, particularly in rural and coastal communities. Small-scale farmers contribute significantly to global aquaculture production, although they often face challenges related to access to credit, training, and markets.

Government support, cooperative models, and sustainable certification schemes are vital in promoting equitable growth and responsible practices in the sector.In conclusion, aquaculture systems and practices have evolved from traditional pond-based operations to sophisticated, technology-driven production systems capable of meeting the growing global demand for aquatic food. The diversity of aquaculture methods—from extensive to intensive, from monoculture to integrated systems—reflects the adaptability of the field to varying ecological and economic contexts. Sustainable aquaculture development requires a balanced approach that integrates productivity, environmental stewardship, animal welfare, and social equity. As innovations continue to emerge, aquaculture holds immense potential to contribute to global nutrition, economic resilience, and ecological sustainability in the decades to come.

1.2 IMPORTANCE OF FISH HEALTH MANAGEMENT

Fish health management is an essential component of sustainable aquaculture, directly influencing productivity, profitability, and environmental balance. As aquaculture continues to expand to meet the global demand for fish and aquatic products, maintaining optimal fish health has become both a biological and economic necessity. Fish health management encompasses all preventive, diagnostic, and therapeutic measures aimed at ensuring the well-being of cultured species and minimizing the impact of diseases. It involves an integrated approach that combines environmental management, nutrition, biosecurity, and disease surveillance. The importance of fish health management extends beyond the survival of cultured species—it determines the overall success and sustainability of the aquaculture industry.

In aquaculture systems, fish are often reared in high densities, which creates a favorable environment for the spread of infectious diseases. Unlike natural ecosystems, where fish populations are dispersed and exposed to a variety of environmental conditions, aquaculture systems confine fish within a controlled but limited space. This confinement, combined with environmental stressors such as poor water quality, inadequate nutrition, or sudden temperature fluctuations, can weaken the immune system of fish, making them more susceptible to infections. Diseases can spread rapidly within such systems, causing massive mortalities in a short period. Effective fish health management seeks to prevent such outbreaks through early detection, preventive measures, and timely intervention.The economic implications of poor fish health are significant. Disease outbreaks can lead to severe production losses, reduced growth rates, increased feed conversion ratios, and even total crop failure. For example, viral and bacterial diseases such as Infectious Hematopoietic Necrosis (IHN), Viral Nervous Necrosis (VNN), and Aeromonas infections have caused billions of dollars in losses globally. In shrimp farming, diseases like White Spot Syndrome Virus (WSSV) and Early Mortality Syndrome (EMS) have devastated aquaculture industries in Asia and Latin America. Beyond direct financial losses, disease outbreaks also result in reduced market access due to trade restrictions, damaged farmer livelihoods, and consumer distrust. Hence, maintaining fish health is crucial not only for individual farmers but also for the stability and growth of the entire aquaculture sector.

Fish health management also has a direct impact on **food security and nutrition**. Fish and other aquatic products are rich sources of high-quality protein, omega-3 fatty acids, vitamins, and minerals essential for human health. As capture fisheries reach their natural limits, aquaculture plays a vital role in supplying affordable and nutritious food to the global population. Disease outbreaks that reduce aquaculture yields can lead to food shortages and increased prices, particularly in developing countries where fish is a staple source of animal protein. Therefore, maintaining fish health contributes to ensuring a consistent and safe food supply, supporting both nutritional security and economic development.From an **environmental perspective**, sound fish health management promotes sustainability and ecosystem stability. Healthy fish populations utilize feed more efficiently, produce less waste, and exhibit better growth performance, reducing the environmental footprint of aquaculture. Conversely, disease outbreaks can lead to overuse of antibiotics and chemicals, which may result in antimicrobial resistance, water pollution, and disruption of natural microbial communities. Proper management practices, including biosecurity measures, vaccination programs, and responsible use of therapeutics, help mitigate these risks. Moreover, effective health management reduces the risk of pathogen spillover from aquaculture facilities into wild fish populations, protecting biodiversity and ecological balance.

Another critical dimension of fish health management is **animal welfare**. As sentient organisms, fish respond physiologically and behaviorally to stress, pain, and poor environmental conditions. Ensuring the welfare of cultured fish through good health practices aligns with ethical standards and growing consumer awareness of sustainable and humane food production. Stress minimization through proper handling, transportation, and water quality management enhances immune function and disease resistance. Welfare-friendly practices are also increasingly becoming prerequisites for eco-certification and market access in international trade. Thus, maintaining fish health not only improves productivity but also supports ethical aquaculture practices.A comprehensive fish health management program integrates **preventive and curative strategies**. Preventive measures are the cornerstone of effective management, as they are more cost-efficient and sustainable than treating diseases after they occur. These include biosecurity protocols, water quality management, proper nutrition, and vaccination. Biosecurity involves controlling the movement of fish, equipment, and personnel to prevent pathogen introduction and spread. Quarantine procedures for new stock, disinfection of tools and tanks, and controlled access to facilities are standard practices. Regular monitoring of water parameters—such as dissolved oxygen, temperature, pH, and ammonia—is essential, as suboptimal conditions can stress fish and predispose them to disease. Nutritionally balanced diets rich in essential vitamins, minerals, and immune-enhancing components like probiotics and prebiotics also play a vital role in promoting resistance to pathogens.

Vaccination and immunoprophylaxis have emerged as powerful tools in fish health management. Vaccines stimulate the immune system to recognize and combat specific pathogens, reducing disease incidence and minimizing the need for antibiotics. For instance, vaccines against bacterial diseases such as *Aeromonas salmonicida* (furunculosis) and *Vibrio anguillarum* (vibriosis) have significantly reduced mortality rates in salmon farming. Continuous research is expanding vaccine availability for a broader range of species and pathogens. Alongside conventional vaccines, novel immunostimulants and natural plant-based therapeutics are being developed to enhance fish immunity and promote sustainable disease prevention.

Disease diagnosis and surveillance are equally important components of fish health management. Early and accurate detection of diseases enables timely intervention and prevents large-scale losses. Diagnostic techniques range from clinical observation and microscopy to advanced molecular tools such as polymerase chain reaction (PCR) and enzyme-linked immunosorbent assay (ELISA). Establishing fish health laboratories and surveillance networks helps monitor emerging pathogens, track disease trends, and support evidence-based management decisions. Data sharing among farmers, veterinarians, and government agencies enhances collective disease control efforts at regional and national levels.The **role of management and education** in fish health cannot be overstated. Farmers, technicians, and hatchery operators need adequate training to identify early signs of disease, understand biosecurity protocols, and implement best management practices. Extension services, workshops, and government-supported training programs are crucial for capacity building, especially in small-scale and developing aquaculture sectors. A knowledgeable workforce is better equipped to maintain healthy production systems, thereby reducing dependency on chemical treatments and enhancing overall sustainability.**Policy and regulatory frameworks** further reinforce fish health management. Governments and international organizations have developed guidelines for aquatic animal health to ensure safe trade and prevent the spread of transboundary diseases. The World Organisation for Animal Health (WOAH, formerly OIE) provides international standards for disease reporting and biosecurity. National regulations on drug usage, waste management, and certification help maintain product safety and environmental integrity. Strengthening institutional coordination between fisheries departments, veterinary services, and research institutions is vital for implementing effective health management systems.

In recent years, **technological advancements** have enhanced the precision and efficiency of fish health management. Automated water quality monitoring systems, artificial intelligence-based disease prediction models, and mobile diagnostic tools allow real-time health assessment and rapid response. Genomic and microbiome research is improving understanding of host-pathogen interactions and leading to the development of more targeted interventions. Such innovations are crucial for addressing the challenges posed by climate change, which is altering disease dynamics through changes in water temperature, salinity, and ecosystem stability.fish health management is the foundation of successful aquaculture. It ensures optimal productivity, economic viability, environmental sustainability, and animal welfare. The consequences of neglecting fish health are far-reaching, affecting not only farmers but also consumers, ecosystems, and global food systems. A proactive and integrated approach—combining preventive strategies, effective diagnostics, responsible therapeutics, and continuous education—offers the best path toward sustainable aquaculture development. As the industry evolves, strengthening fish health management will remain central to achieving a resilient and responsible aquaculture sector capable of meeting the nutritional and economic needs of a growing global population.

1.3 ECONOMIC AND ECOLOGICAL IMPACT OF FISH DISEASES

Fish diseases represent one of the most significant challenges facing global aquaculture today, with far-reaching economic, ecological, and social consequences. As aquaculture has evolved into a major contributor to global food security, accounting for over half of the world's fish supply, the occurrence and spread of diseases have emerged as critical threats to productivity and sustainability. The impacts of fish diseases are multidimensional—extending beyond the immediate mortality of aquatic animals to affect livelihoods, trade, food availability, and the stability of aquatic ecosystems. Understanding the economic and ecological repercussions of fish diseases is essential for developing effective management, preventive, and policy strategies to ensure the long-term resilience of aquaculture systems.

From an **economic standpoint**, fish diseases can cause devastating financial losses at both micro and macro levels. At the farm level, disease outbreaks often lead to massive mortalities, reduced growth rates, and lower feed efficiency. This translates directly into decreased yields, higher production costs, and reduced profitability. For instance, farmers may face expenses related to the purchase of medications, disinfectants, diagnostic services, and water treatment systems. Furthermore, preventive measures such as vaccination programs, quarantine facilities, and biosecurity infrastructure add to operational costs. While these investments are crucial, they can be burdensome for small-scale farmers who lack financial resources. The cumulative result is reduced competitiveness and, in some cases, the collapse of local aquaculture enterprises.

Globally, the **economic losses due to fish diseases** are staggering. It is estimated that disease outbreaks cause billions of dollars in losses each year. For example, viral diseases such as White Spot Syndrome Virus (WSSV) in shrimp, Infectious Salmon Anemia (ISA) in salmon, and Koi Herpesvirus (KHV) in carp have led to catastrophic losses in major aquaculture-producing countries. The 1990s outbreak of ISA in Chile's salmon industry resulted in a decline of over 75% in production and billions in economic losses. Similarly, the outbreak of Early Mortality Syndrome (EMS) in shrimp farms across Southeast Asia during the 2010s caused widespread collapse of shrimp aquaculture, leading to massive job losses and market shortages. These examples underscore how a single pathogenic event can disrupt entire industries and economies.

In addition to direct production losses, **indirect economic impacts** also play a significant role. Disease outbreaks often lead to trade restrictions and loss of export markets due to biosecurity concerns. Countries importing aquatic products demand strict health certification and compliance with international sanitary standards. When an exporting nation experiences a disease outbreak, it may face trade bans or reduced demand, leading to economic isolation and loss of foreign exchange earnings. For example, the presence of pathogens such as *Vibrio cholerae* or *Mycobacterium marinum* in aquaculture products can trigger import restrictions in major markets like the European Union or the United States. The resultant trade disruptions can severely affect national economies, particularly in developing countries where aquaculture is a vital source of income and employment.

Fish diseases also exert **social and livelihood impacts**, especially in rural and coastal communities dependent on aquaculture for sustenance and income. Disease-induced production losses often force small-scale farmers into debt, leading to socioeconomic instability. Reduced income limits access to education, healthcare, and food security, exacerbating poverty cycles. Furthermore, women—who play significant roles in aquaculture processing and marketing—are disproportionately affected by reduced production and employment opportunities. The ripple effect of aquaculture disease outbreaks thus extends beyond the farm gate, influencing the well-being of entire communities.

Beyond economics, the **ecological impact of fish diseases** is equally profound. Aquatic ecosystems are highly interconnected, and pathogens can move freely between cultured and wild populations. Disease outbreaks in aquaculture facilities may spill over into natural water bodies, affecting native species and biodiversity. For example, the spread of Infectious Salmon Anemia and sea lice (*Lepeophtheirus salmonis*) from salmon farms to wild salmon populations has been documented in Norway, Scotland, and Canada, leading to population declines and ecological imbalances. Similarly, Koi Herpesvirus (KHV) outbreaks in farmed carp have been linked to mortality events in wild carp populations, disrupting local ecosystems.

The **introduction of exotic pathogens** through international trade and the translocation of live fish also poses ecological risks. Globalization of the aquaculture industry has facilitated the movement of species across borders, sometimes without adequate health screening. This has led to the introduction of novel pathogens into new environments where native species have little or no immunity. For instance, the introduction of the parasite *Gyrodactylus salaris* to Norwegian rivers through infected salmon stocks resulted in the near extinction of local salmon populations. Similarly, *Aphanomyces invadans*, the causative agent of Epizootic Ulcerative Syndrome (EUS), has spread across Asia, Africa, and Australia, infecting numerous freshwater and estuarine fish species. Such outbreaks highlight how inadequate biosecurity measures can have devastating consequences for natural biodiversity and ecosystem functioning.

Fish diseases can also disrupt **trophic dynamics and ecological balance** within aquatic environments. Diseased fish often exhibit behavioral changes such as reduced feeding or erratic swimming, making them more susceptible to predation. This alters predator-prey relationships and can lead to cascading ecological effects. Large-scale fish mortalities, particularly in enclosed water bodies, result in organic matter accumulation and oxygen depletion, causing eutrophication and deterioration of water quality. The decomposition of dead fish releases nitrogen and phosphorus into the water, promoting algal blooms that further degrade habitat quality and threaten other aquatic life forms.

Climate change further exacerbates the ecological and economic impact of fish diseases. Rising water temperatures, salinity shifts, and changes in rainfall patterns can stress aquatic organisms and alter pathogen dynamics. Warmer conditions often accelerate pathogen replication and extend the transmission season, increasing the frequency and severity of outbreaks. For instance, Vibrio-related infections in marine fish and shellfish have become more prevalent in temperate regions due to rising sea surface temperatures. Climate-induced disease emergence poses new challenges for both farmed and wild fish populations, demanding adaptive management strategies and enhanced disease surveillance systems.To mitigate these economic and ecological consequences, **integrated fish health management and biosecurity** are indispensable. Preventive strategies such as vaccination, water quality control, quarantine, and health certification of seed stock can significantly reduce disease incidence. Early detection and rapid response systems help minimize economic losses and prevent pathogen spread. At the policy level, national and international collaboration through organizations such as the World Organisation for Animal Health (WOAH) and the Food and Agriculture Organization (FAO) is essential for harmonizing disease control standards and ensuring safe trade.

CHAPTER 2:

ETIOLOGY AND CLASSIFICATION OF FISH DISEASES

2.1 ETIOLOGY AND CLASSIFICATION OF FISH DISEASES

Fish diseases arise from a wide range of causes, generally categorized into **infectious** and **non-infectious** types. Understanding the distinction between these categories, along with their specific etiological agents, is fundamental for diagnosis, prevention, and control. In aquaculture systems, where fish are reared in dense populations and under controlled conditions, disease outbreaks can occur rapidly and spread extensively, making comprehensive knowledge of disease etiology crucial for effective management and sustainability.**Infectious diseases** are caused by pathogenic microorganisms such as bacteria, viruses, fungi, or parasites that can invade, multiply, and cause damage to the host. These diseases are transmissible, spreading directly through water, contact, contaminated equipment, or carriers like wild fish, invertebrates, and humans. In aquaculture, infectious diseases represent the most significant threat due to their potential to cause high mortality and rapid transmission within confined systems. The severity of infection depends on the virulence of the pathogen, the susceptibility of the host, and environmental conditions. Poor water quality, overcrowding, stress, and nutritional deficiencies can compromise the fish immune system, increasing vulnerability to pathogens. Common examples include *Aeromonas hydrophila* (bacterial hemorrhagic septicemia), *Ichthyophthirius multifiliis* (white spot disease), and Koi Herpesvirus (KHV) infection.

Non-infectious diseases, on the other hand, are caused by factors that are not transmissible between individuals. These may include environmental stressors (such as poor water quality, oxygen depletion, or toxic substances), nutritional imbalances, genetic abnormalities, or physical injuries. Non-infectious diseases often predispose fish to secondary infections by weakening their immune defenses. For instance, exposure to high levels of ammonia or nitrite can cause gill damage, leading to respiratory distress and increased susceptibility to opportunistic bacterial infections. Similarly, vitamin C deficiency may result in skeletal deformities and poor wound healing, indirectly affecting survival rates. Unlike infectious diseases, non-infectious conditions can be mitigated effectively through improved management practices, water quality control, and balanced nutrition.

2.2 CLASSIFICATION OF FISH DISEASES

Fish diseases can be broadly classified based on the nature of their causative agents. The primary categories include **bacterial, viral, fungal, parasitic, nutritional, and environmental** diseases. Each group has distinct characteristics, modes of transmission, and management strategies.

1. **Bacterial Diseases:**

   Bacterial infections are among the most common and economically significant diseases in aquaculture. They can be caused by both gram-negative and gram-positive bacteria, many of which are opportunistic pathogens present in the aquatic environment. Common bacterial diseases include *Aeromonas hydrophila* (motile Aeromonas septicemia), *Vibrio anguillarum* (vibriosis), *Edwardsiella tarda* (edwardsiellosis), and *Flavobacterium columnare* (columnaris disease). Symptoms often include hemorrhages, ulcers, fin rot, exophthalmia, and internal organ necrosis. Transmission occurs through waterborne exposure, direct contact, or contaminated equipment. Effective control measures involve maintaining good water quality, vaccination, antibiotic therapy under veterinary supervision, and biosecurity management.

2. **Viral Diseases:**

   Viral infections are highly contagious and can cause severe mortality, especially in intensive aquaculture systems. They are often species-specific and difficult to treat, as antiviral therapies are limited. Examples include Koi Herpesvirus Disease (KHVD) in carp, Infectious Salmon Anemia Virus (ISAV) in salmon, Infectious Pancreatic Necrosis Virus (IPNV) in trout, and White Spot Syndrome Virus (WSSV) in shrimp. Clinical signs may include lethargy, abnormal swimming, pale gills, and hemorrhages. Since no direct cure exists, management focuses on prevention through biosecurity, disinfection, and vaccination where available. Viral diseases have significant implications for international trade and biosecurity due to their potential for rapid, transboundary spread.

3. **Fungal Diseases:**

Fungal infections typically occur as secondary invaders following injury or stress, though some species are primary pathogens. Common fungal diseases include *Saprolegniasis*, caused by *Saprolegnia* species, and *Branchiomycosis* (gill rot) caused by *Branchiomyces demigrans*. Affected fish often exhibit cotton-like growths on the skin, gills, or eggs, leading to tissue necrosis and impaired respiration. Fungal spores are ubiquitous in aquatic environments and thrive under conditions of poor hygiene, low temperature, or organic pollution. Management involves improving water quality, using antifungal treatments (such as formalin or potassium permanganate under guidance), and preventing injuries.

4. **Parasitic Diseases:**

Parasites are major contributors to morbidity and mortality in aquaculture, ranging from microscopic protozoans to macroscopic crustaceans. Protozoan parasites such as *Ichthyophthirius multifiliis* (white spot or ich) and *Trichodina* spp. cause external infestations, while *Myxobolus cerebralis* (whirling disease) and *Eimeria* spp. may affect internal organs. Metazoan parasites, including monogeneans like *Gyrodactylus* and crustaceans such as *Lernaea* (anchor worm) and *Argulus* (fish louse), can cause tissue damage, secondary bacterial infections, and growth retardation. Control measures include chemical treatments, quarantine, and integrated parasite management through biological control and improved sanitation.

5. **Nutritional Diseases:**

Nutritional imbalances can lead to various health problems, often manifesting as growth retardation, deformities, and reduced reproductive performance. Deficiencies in essential vitamins, minerals, amino acids, or fatty acids may cause specific syndromes—for example, vitamin C deficiency results in skeletal deformities, while vitamin E deficiency leads to muscular dystrophy. Poor-quality or imbalanced feed can also suppress immune function, increasing susceptibility to infectious diseases. Ensuring nutritionally balanced diets, proper feed storage, and feeding management are vital to preventing such disorders.

2.3 EMERGING AND TRANSBOUNDARY AQUATIC PATHOGENS

In recent decades, the aquaculture industry has witnessed the emergence of **novel and transboundary aquatic pathogens**, posing serious challenges to fish health and trade. Emerging diseases are often linked to globalization, intensified production, climate change, and the translocation of live aquatic organisms. These factors facilitate the spread of pathogens across geographical boundaries and between wild and cultured fish populations.One of the most devastating examples is the **White Spot Syndrome Virus (WSSV)** in shrimp, first identified in Asia and later spreading worldwide. Similarly, **Tilapia Lake Virus (TiLV)** has recently emerged as a major threat to global tilapia production, affecting countries across Asia, Africa, and Latin America. Other transboundary diseases include **Infectious Salmon Anemia (ISA)**, **Koi Herpesvirus (KHV)**, and **Epizootic Ulcerative Syndrome (EUS)**. These pathogens have caused substantial economic losses, trade restrictions, and ecological disturbances.The **drivers of disease emergence** are multifactorial. High stocking densities and genetic uniformity in farmed populations increase vulnerability to infectious agents. Climate change alters water temperature and salinity, influencing pathogen virulence and host susceptibility. International trade and movement of broodstock without proper quarantine procedures introduce new pathogens to previously unaffected regions. Moreover, the use of untreated effluents and open-water culture systems facilitates disease transmission to wild populations.Addressing emerging and transboundary diseases requires **international cooperation, biosecurity, and surveillance**. The World Organisation for Animal Health (WOAH) and the Food and Agriculture Organization (FAO) have developed guidelines for monitoring, reporting, and controlling aquatic animal diseases. Quarantine protocols, health certification, and early warning systems are critical to preventing pathogen introduction and spread. Research into vaccine development, host genetics, and pathogen ecology further contributes to effective long-term control.strategies.

CHAPTER 3:

ANATOMY AND PHYSIOLOGY OF FISH RELEVANT TO DISEASE

3.1 IMMUNE SYSTEM OF FISH

The immune system of fish plays a vital role in maintaining health, preventing disease, and ensuring survival in diverse aquatic environments. As the first vertebrates to possess both innate and adaptive immune mechanisms, fish provide an important evolutionary bridge in understanding the vertebrate immune system. Their immune responses are shaped by environmental factors such as water temperature, salinity, and the presence of pathogens, making immunity in fish a dynamic and complex process. In aquaculture, knowledge of fish immunology is essential for developing disease prevention strategies, designing vaccines, and enhancing resistance through improved nutrition and management.

Fish, like other vertebrates, possess two major components of the immune system: **innate (non-specific) immunity** and **adaptive (specific) immunity**. These systems interact closely to recognize, respond to, and eliminate invading pathogens. The innate immune system provides the first line of defense and operates rapidly, while the adaptive system offers specific, long-term protection following exposure to antigens. Together, these mechanisms form an integrated network that maintains homeostasis and protects against microbial infections, parasites, and environmental stressors.The innate immune system in fish is the **primary defense mechanism** that operates immediately upon pathogen exposure. It includes **physical barriers, cellular defenses, and humoral factors**.The skin, scales, and mucous layers serve as the first line of defense. The **mucus** secreted by epithelial cells contains antimicrobial peptides, lysozymes, lectins, and immunoglobulins that inhibit microbial colonization. The mucus also physically traps pathogens and helps in their removal. The **gills**, while serving respiratory functions, are also key immune organs as they are constantly exposed to waterborne pathogens. Mucosal surfaces in gills and intestines contain immune cells that recognize and respond to invading microbes. Similarly, the **gut-associated lymphoid tissue (GALT)** forms a critical part of the mucosal immune system, protecting fish from pathogens entering through ingestion.Innate immune cells in fish include

macrophages, neutrophils, monocytes, natural killer (NK)-like cells, and dendritic-like cells. These cells perform phagocytosis, engulfing and destroying pathogens through enzymatic degradation or oxidative mechanisms. **Macrophages** are multifunctional cells responsible for both pathogen destruction and antigen presentation to adaptive immune cells. **Neutrophils** rapidly migrate to infection sites and release reactive oxygen species to kill invading microbes. NK-like cells target virus-infected or abnormal cells, contributing to antiviral defense. The innate immune cells are regulated by signaling molecules known as **cytokines**, which coordinate the inflammatory response and activate other immune components.Several soluble molecules play critical roles in the fish innate immune response. **Lysozyme**, an enzyme found in mucus, serum, and tissues, degrades bacterial cell walls, particularly those of Gram-positive bacteria. **Complement proteins** constitute another major component, acting in a cascade to opsonize pathogens, enhance phagocytosis, and cause cell lysis. The **complement system** in fish consists of classical, alternative, and lectin pathways, similar to those in higher vertebrates. **C-reactive proteins, lectins, transferrin, and antimicrobial peptides** also participate in pathogen recognition and neutralization. Together, these mechanisms form an effective barrier against a wide range of infections before the adaptive immune system is activated.

Adaptive (Specific) Immune System

The adaptive immune system in fish provides **specific and long-lasting protection** against pathogens. Although less complex than that of mammals, it exhibits key features such as antigen recognition, immunological memory, and clonal expansion of lymphocytes.Fish lack bone marrow and lymph nodes but possess several primary and secondary lymphoid organs that perform analogous functions.

- The **thymus** is the primary site for T-cell development and differentiation. It is located dorsally near the gill cavity and is active in young fish, decreasing in size with age.
- The **head kidney (pronephros)** serves as the major hematopoietic and immune organ in teleost fish, producing lymphocytes, macrophages, and granulocytes. It also plays a crucial role in antigen processing and antibody production.
- The **spleen** functions as a secondary lymphoid organ involved in antigen trapping, lymphocyte activation, and antibody synthesis.

- The **mucosa-associated lymphoid tissues** in gills, skin, and gut serve as local defense sites against mucosal pathogens.

Cell-mediated immune responses are primarily mediated by **T lymphocytes**, which develop in the thymus. Fish possess T-cell subsets analogous to mammalian helper T cells (Th) and cytotoxic T cells (Tc). **Helper T cells (Th)** secrete cytokines that regulate immune responses, activate macrophages, and assist B cells in antibody production. **Cytotoxic T cells (Tc)** directly kill infected cells by releasing perforins and granzymes. The presence of major histocompatibility complex (MHC) molecules in fish facilitates antigen presentation and T-cell activation, though the diversity of MHC genes varies among species.Humoral immunity in fish is mediated by **B lymphocytes** and **antibodies (immunoglobulins)**. Upon encountering an antigen, B cells differentiate into plasma cells that secrete antibodies specific to the pathogen. Teleost fish produce three main classes of immunoglobulins: **IgM, IgD, and IgT (or IgZ)**.

- **IgM** is the most abundant antibody in serum and plays a major role in systemic immune responses.
- **IgD** is less understood but is thought to participate in immune regulation.
- **IgT/IgZ** is primarily involved in mucosal immunity, especially in gut, gill, and skin surfaces.

  The presence of these antibodies provides specificity to the immune response and forms the basis for immunological memory. Upon re-exposure to the same pathogen, the response is faster and more robust—a principle utilized in fish vaccination programs.

Mucosal Immunity

Mucosal immunity is a critical aspect of fish defense since mucosal tissues (skin, gills, and intestines) are constantly exposed to pathogens. The **mucosa-associated lymphoid tissue (MALT)** includes **GALT (gut-associated), GIALT (gill-associated), and SALT (skin-associated)** lymphoid tissues. These structures contain immune cells capable of recognizing antigens, producing antibodies, and initiating localized immune responses. Mucosal immunity plays a major role in protecting fish against waterborne infections, particularly in aquaculture environments where exposure to pathogens is continuous. Mucosal vaccines are increasingly being developed to stimulate these localized immune defenses effectively.Cytokines are signaling proteins that mediate communication between immune cells. In fish, cytokines such as **interleukins (ILs), interferons (IFNs), tumor necrosis factors (TNFs), and transforming growth factors (TGFs)** have been identified and characterized. **Interferons** play key roles in antiviral defense by inducing the expression of antiviral proteins, while **TNF-α** and **IL-1β** promote inflammation and phagocyte activation. The balance between pro-inflammatory and anti-inflammatory cytokines determines the intensity and duration of immune responses. Molecular studies have revealed that many cytokine genes in fish are evolutionarily conserved with those of higher vertebrates, highlighting their fundamental roles in vertebrate immunity.The efficiency of the fish immune system is profoundly influenced by environmental conditions and nutrition. Water temperature, pH, oxygen levels, and pollution can alter immune functions. For instance, low temperatures may suppress antibody production, whereas thermal stress increases susceptibility to pathogens. Nutritional status is equally important—vitamins (A, C, E), minerals (zinc, selenium), fatty acids, and immunostimulants (β-glucans, probiotics) enhance immune responses. Balanced diets not only promote growth but also strengthen resistance against infections. Conversely, malnutrition or feed contamination can weaken immunity and increase disease risk in cultured species.

Applications in Aquaculture

Understanding fish immunology has practical applications in **disease control and vaccination**. Vaccines stimulate adaptive immunity, providing specific protection against bacterial and viral pathogens. The success of vaccination programs against *Vibrio anguillarum*, *Aeromonas salmonicida*, and *Streptococcus iniae* demonstrates the effectiveness of harnessing fish immune responses. Immunostimulants and probiotics are also used to enhance innate defenses, especially in larval and juvenile stages where adaptive immunity is not fully developed. Molecular immunology and genomics are now enabling selective breeding for disease-resistant strains, offering sustainable solutions for aquaculture health management.

3.2 GILLS, SKIN, AND MUCUS AS DEFENSE BARRIERS

The gills, skin, and mucus of fish form the primary **physical and immunological barriers** between the internal body environment and the surrounding aquatic habitat. Together, they constitute the **mucosal defense system**, serving not only as protective structures but also as dynamic components of the fish immune system. These surfaces are continuously exposed to a diverse array of pathogens, including bacteria, viruses, fungi, and parasites, as well as to environmental stressors such as pollutants and temperature fluctuations. Therefore, understanding the protective functions of these tissues is crucial for developing effective health management and disease prevention strategies in aquaculture.

1. The Skin as the First Line of Defense

The **skin of fish** acts as the most extensive barrier against mechanical injury, chemical irritants, and microbial invasion. It is composed of three main layers: the **epidermis, dermis, and hypodermis**, each contributing to both structural integrity and immune protection.The **epidermis** is the outermost layer, consisting of living cells including epidermal cells, mucous (goblet) cells, and specialized immune cells such as Langerhans-like and macrophage-like cells. Unlike terrestrial vertebrates, fish skin lacks keratinization, keeping the surface moist and permeable. The **dermis** lies beneath the epidermis and is composed of collagen and elastin fibers that provide strength and flexibility. Embedded within the dermis are chromatophores for coloration and sensory structures that detect mechanical and chemical changes in the environment. The **hypodermis** connects the skin to underlying musculature and contains blood vessels that facilitate immune cell transport.The skin is an **immunologically active organ**. It is rich in **skin-associated lymphoid tissue (SALT)**, which functions similarly to mammalian mucosa-associated lymphoid tissues. SALT contains immune cells such as macrophages, neutrophils, dendritic-like cells, and lymphocytes that participate in both innate and adaptive immune responses. These cells detect pathogen-associated molecular patterns (PAMPs) through **pattern recognition receptors (PRRs)** like toll-like receptors (TLRs), triggering local inflammatory responses and cytokine secretion. The skin thus serves not only as a physical barrier but also as an **immune surveillance site**, capable of mounting immediate defensive responses against invading microorganisms.Skin damage from handling, crowding, or poor water quality can compromise its barrier function, providing an entry point for pathogens such as *Aeromonas hydrophila* or *Saprolegnia spp.*. Therefore, maintaining skin integrity through optimal husbandry and water conditions is critical for disease prevention in aquaculture. Many ectoparasites, including *Ichthyophthirius multifiliis* (white spot disease), first attach to the skin, making it a major interface for host-pathogen interactions.

2. The Gills as a Respiratory and Immune Interface

The **gills** are multifunctional organs primarily responsible for gas exchange, osmoregulation, and excretion, but they also play a central role in **immunological defense**. Due to their large surface area and direct contact with water, gills are constantly exposed to pathogens, toxins, and suspended particles, making them vulnerable yet critical immune structures.Each gill consists of arches bearing filaments and lamellae, which create an extensive surface area for oxygen and carbon dioxide exchange. The gill epithelium is composed of **chloride cells (ionocytes)**, **pavement cells**, and **mucous cells**, supported by a dense capillary network. The delicate architecture allows efficient gas exchange but also makes the gills one of the most susceptible tissues to infection and environmental damage.The **gill-associated lymphoid tissue (GIALT)** forms a crucial part of the mucosal immune system. GIALT comprises both innate and adaptive immune components. **Macrophages, neutrophils, and lymphocytes** are frequently found in gill tissues, performing immune surveillance and pathogen clearance. Gills produce **antimicrobial peptides (AMPs)** such as defensins and lysozymes, as well as **complement proteins** that neutralize or lyse pathogens. The mucus covering the gill surface contains immunoglobulins, particularly **IgT**, which plays a key role in mucosal immunity.Despite their immune defenses, gills are among the most common entry points for aquatic pathogens. Bacteria such as *Flavobacterium branchiophilum* (bacterial gill disease), viruses such as infectious hematopoietic necrosis virus (IHNV), and parasites such as *Ichthyobodo necator* or *Dactylogyrus spp.* frequently target gill tissues. These infections can lead to epithelial hyperplasia, lamellar fusion, necrosis, and impaired respiration. Poor water quality—especially high ammonia or low dissolved oxygen—exacerbates gill damage, increasing susceptibility to infections. Therefore, **gill health monitoring** is a key component of aquaculture disease management.Fish gills are unique in balancing respiratory efficiency with immune protection. The presence of **tight junctions** between epithelial cells prevents pathogen penetration while maintaining permeability for gas and ion exchange. The **local immune responses** in gills, including cytokine production and leukocyte recruitment, act rapidly upon pathogen recognition. Moreover, mucosal vaccination strategies increasingly target the gills to stimulate site-specific immunity, enhancing disease resistance without the need for invasive administration.

3. Mucus: The Multifunctional Protective Barrier

The **mucus layer** that covers the skin, gills, and other external surfaces serves as a **biochemical and physical shield** against environmental hazards and pathogens. Far from being a passive secretion, fish mucus is a highly complex and dynamic matrix composed of **mucins, enzymes, immunoglobulins, antimicrobial peptides, lysozyme, lectins, and protease inhibitors**.Mucus is secreted primarily by **goblet cells** located in the epidermis and gill epithelia. Its viscosity and composition can change depending on environmental conditions, species, and health status. The main structural component, **mucin glycoproteins**, forms a gel-like network that traps particles and microorganisms. This matrix also contains bioactive molecules such as **lysozyme**, which hydrolyzes bacterial cell walls; **complement proteins**, which opsonize pathogens; and **lectins**, which bind to specific carbohydrate residues on microbial surfaces, facilitating recognition and elimination.Mucus functions as an **immunologically active medium**. It contains **immunoglobulins (mainly IgM and IgT)** that neutralize pathogens before they can invade tissues. The **innate immune molecules**, including proteases, alkaline phosphatases, and antimicrobial peptides, provide immediate defense by destroying or inhibiting microbial growth. In addition, the mucus harbors beneficial microbial communities (the **mucosal microbiome**) that compete with pathogens, producing antimicrobial substances and modulating host immunity. Disruption of this microbial balance, often due to antibiotic overuse or poor water quality, can increase disease susceptibility.Mucus secretion often increases during stress or infection, forming a thicker protective layer. While this response can be beneficial, excessive mucus production can interfere with respiration and osmoregulation, especially on gill surfaces. The composition of mucus also changes under disease conditions; for example, elevated levels of lysozyme and protease activity have been observed during bacterial infections, indicating activation of immune defenses. Analysis of mucus components is increasingly used as a **non-invasive diagnostic tool** for assessing fish health in aquaculture.In intensive aquaculture systems, maintaining mucus integrity is critical. Factors such as rough handling, net abrasion, poor water quality, and chemical exposure can damage mucus layers, compromising immunity. The use of immunostimulants, probiotics, and dietary supplements (e.g., β-glucans, vitamins, and trace minerals) has been shown to enhance mucus production and improve its antimicrobial properties. Moreover, the development of **mucosal vaccines** aims to stimulate immune responses directly within mucus-associated tissues, providing localized and long-lasting protection against pathogens.

4. Integrated Function of Gills, Skin, and Mucus in Immunity

The gills, skin, and mucus do not act independently; rather, they function as an **integrated defense system** that provides both mechanical protection and immunological resistance. Together, these tissues form the **first line of defense** against infections, collectively known as the **mucosal immune system**. When pathogens breach the mucus layer, immune cells within the skin or gills rapidly respond through phagocytosis, cytokine secretion, and antibody production. This local response can also trigger systemic immunity through signaling pathways involving lymphoid organs such as the head kidney and spleen.The coordination among these barriers ensures that pathogens are neutralized early, minimizing tissue damage and maintaining physiological balance. The effectiveness of this system, however, depends heavily on environmental quality, nutritional status, and genetic resilience of the fish.The gills, skin, and mucus of fish represent sophisticated biological interfaces that combine physical, chemical, and immunological defenses. They not only protect against pathogenic invasion but also play vital roles in respiration, osmoregulation, and communication with the external environment. Their effectiveness determines the overall health and disease resistance of fish, particularly in aquaculture systems where stress and pathogen exposure are constant challenges. Maintaining the integrity of these barriers through proper management, nutrition, and environmental control is essential for sustainable aquaculture production. Future research focusing on enhancing mucosal immunity, microbiome modulation, and targeted vaccination will further strengthen disease prevention strategies, ensuring the health and productivity of cultured fish species.

3.3 STRESS PHYSIOLOGY AND SUSCEPTIBILITY TO DISEASES

Stress is an inevitable part of the aquatic environment and plays a significant role in the overall health and disease resistance of fish. In aquaculture, stress is particularly critical because cultured fish are often exposed to artificial conditions, including crowding, handling, poor water quality, and transportation. Although short-term or acute stress can sometimes stimulate adaptive physiological responses, chronic or prolonged stress impairs immune function, growth, and reproduction, leading to increased vulnerability to diseases. Understanding the **physiology of stress and its relationship to disease susceptibility** is, therefore, essential for effective fish health management and sustainable aquaculture operations.

1. Concept of Stress in Fish

Stress in fish can be defined as a **physiological condition resulting from environmental or internal disturbances that threaten homeostasis**. The concept of homeostasis refers to the body's ability to maintain stable internal conditions despite external fluctuations. When fish encounter a stressor—whether physical, chemical, biological, or social—they respond through a series of neuroendocrine, metabolic, and immunological adjustments aimed at restoring balance. These responses are mediated primarily by the **hypothalamus–pituitary–interrenal (HPI) axis**, which is functionally equivalent to the hypothalamus–pituitary–adrenal (HPA) axis in mammals.stressors in aquaculture are numerous and can be categorized as **acute** (short-term, such as netting or transport) or **chronic** (long-term, such as poor water quality or high stocking density). While acute stress may temporarily enhance alertness and immune readiness, chronic stress causes physiological exhaustion, immunosuppression, and metabolic imbalances, which predispose fish to disease outbreaks.

2. The Stress Response Mechanism

When a fish perceives a stressor, its response unfolds in **three interrelated phases**: the **primary**, **secondary**, and **tertiary** responses.This phase involves **neuroendocrine activation**, primarily of the HPI axis. The hypothalamus releases corticotropin-releasing hormone (CRH), which stimulates the pituitary gland to secrete adrenocorticotropic hormone (ACTH). ACTH, in turn, acts on the **interrenal cells** located in the head kidney to release **cortisol**, the principal stress hormone in fish. Cortisol mobilizes energy reserves by increasing glucose production, ensuring that the organism has sufficient energy to cope with stress. At the same time, the **sympathetic–chromaffin system (SCS)** releases catecholamines such as adrenaline and noradrenaline, which increase heart rate, blood pressure, and oxygen uptake, preparing the fish for immediate action.This phase includes a wide range of **metabolic, hematological, and osmoregulatory changes**. Elevated cortisol levels lead to hyperglycemia (increased blood glucose), altered ion balance, and changes in oxygen consumption. There is often a reduction in plasma protein levels and an increase in lactate, indicating anaerobic metabolism during stress. Prolonged cortisol exposure can impair growth by diverting energy from anabolic processes such as protein synthesis to catabolic processes. Osmoregulation, an essential function for aquatic organisms, is disrupted under stress, leading to ionic imbalances and increased permeability of gill and skin epithelia. These physiological disturbances compromise overall fitness and reduce the ability of fish to respond to pathogens effectively.This phase reflects the **whole-animal or population-level consequences** of prolonged stress, including reduced growth, poor feed conversion, altered behavior, suppressed reproduction, and heightened disease susceptibility. Chronic stress can lead to increased mortality rates, either directly through physiological exhaustion or indirectly through opportunistic infections that exploit weakened immune defenses.

3. Stress and the Immune System

One of the most significant consequences of stress in fish is **immunosuppression**, which increases the likelihood of disease. The relationship between stress and immunity is complex, involving both **hormonal regulation** and **cellular responses**.Cortisol is a potent immunomodulatory hormone. While short-term increases may enhance certain innate immune functions (such as leukocyte activation), chronic elevation leads to immunosuppression. Cortisol reduces the number and activity of lymphocytes, suppresses antibody production, and inhibits cytokine synthesis. It also diminishes the activity of phagocytes, reducing their ability to engulf and destroy pathogens. As a result, prolonged stress decreases both **innate and adaptive immune responses**, rendering fish more susceptible to bacterial, viral, and parasitic infections.The innate immune system provides the first line of defense against pathogens, and its components—such as macrophages, neutrophils, lysozyme, and complement proteins—are directly affected by stress. Studies have shown that exposure to chronic stressors such as poor water quality or crowding reduces phagocytic activity and lysozyme levels in fish. Moreover, oxidative stress, a byproduct of prolonged stress, damages immune cells and reduces their functionality.Adaptive immunity, mediated by T and B lymphocytes, is also compromised under stress. Elevated cortisol levels inhibit lymphocyte proliferation and antibody production, weakening the humoral immune response. This immunosuppression leads to lower vaccine efficacy in stressed fish populations, underscoring the importance of minimizing stress before and after vaccination in aquaculture.

4. Stress-Induced Disease Susceptibility

The link between stress and disease susceptibility is well documented across aquaculture species. Stress creates physiological conditions that favor **pathogen invasion and proliferation**. For instance, stress-induced skin or gill damage compromises physical barriers, while immunosuppression provides an opportunity for opportunistic pathogens to thrive.Fish under stress are more prone to bacterial diseases such as **Aeromoniasis** (*Aeromonas hydrophila*), **Vibriosis** (*Vibrio spp.*), and **Columnaris disease** (*Flavobacterium columnare*). These pathogens are often present in the environment but only cause disease when host defenses are weakened.Stressful conditions such as poor water quality or overcrowding also favor parasitic infestations like *Ichthyophthirius multifiliis* and *Dactylogyrus spp.*, as well as fungal infections caused by *Saprolegnia spp.* The increased production of stress-related mucus provides a nutrient-rich substrate for pathogen colonization.Stress has been implicated in outbreaks of viral infections such as infectious pancreatic necrosis (IPN) and koi herpesvirus disease (KHVD). The reactivation of latent viral infections under stress conditions mirrors similar phenomena observed in higher vertebrates, where stress hormones suppress antiviral defenses.

5. Environmental and Managerial Stressors in Aquaculture

In aquaculture, stress can result from multiple operational factors:

- **Water Quality Stressors:** Fluctuations in temperature, dissolved oxygen, pH, salinity, ammonia, and nitrite levels are major contributors to chronic stress.
- **Handling and Transportation:** Netting, grading, and transport cause acute stress, elevating cortisol and glucose levels within minutes.
- **Stocking Density:** Overcrowding leads to social stress, competition for resources, and increased aggression, elevating stress hormone levels.
- **Poor Nutrition:** Nutrient deficiencies weaken the immune system and reduce stress tolerance.
- **Pollution and Chemicals:** Pesticides, heavy metals, and disinfectants disrupt endocrine and immune systems, increasing disease risk.

CHAPTER 4:

ENVIRONMENTAL FACTORS AFFECTING FISH HEALTH

4.1 WATER QUALITY PARAMETERS (DO, PH, TEMPERATURE, AMMONIA)

Water quality is the cornerstone of successful aquaculture. It not only influences the physiological performance and survival of cultured fish but also determines the overall health and productivity of the aquatic system. Unlike terrestrial animals, fish are completely surrounded by their environment, and thus, even minor fluctuations in water parameters can have profound effects on their metabolism, immune response, and disease resistance. Among the most critical water quality parameters are **dissolved oxygen (DO), pH, temperature, and ammonia concentration**. These four factors are interdependent and together define the quality and stability of the aquatic habitat. Maintaining optimal levels of these parameters is essential to prevent stress, enhance growth, and reduce disease outbreaks in aquaculture systems.

Dissolved oxygen (DO) refers to the amount of free, non-compound oxygen present in water, available for respiration by aquatic organisms. It is one of the most vital water quality parameters, as oxygen is required for aerobic metabolism, energy production, and overall physiological function.Fish extract oxygen from water through their gills. Adequate DO levels are essential for efficient respiration, nutrient assimilation, and waste metabolism. Oxygen supports key biochemical processes, including cellular respiration, immune function, and reproduction. Low DO conditions, or **hypoxia**, impair aerobic metabolism, forcing fish to shift to anaerobic pathways that generate lactic acid and energy inefficiently. Prolonged oxygen deficiency can lead to tissue damage, metabolic acidosis, and death.

Several factors affect DO concentration, including temperature, salinity, water turbulence, photosynthetic activity, and organic loading. **Colder water holds more oxygen**, whereas oxygen solubility decreases as temperature increases. **Eutrophication** from excessive nutrient input stimulates algal blooms that initially increase DO during daylight through photosynthesis but cause severe depletion at night when respiration dominates. High levels of organic matter from uneaten feed and feces also consume oxygen during decomposition.For most freshwater fish, a **DO concentration above 5 mg/L** is considered optimal for growth and health. Concentrations below

3 mg/L are stressful, and levels under 1–2 mg/L can be fatal, particularly for sensitive species like trout. Maintaining adequate aeration through diffusers, paddlewheels, or mechanical aerators is therefore crucial in aquaculture systems, especially in high-density ponds and recirculating setups.Chronic low oxygen levels suppress feeding, reduce growth rates, and weaken immune defenses. Hypoxia impairs macrophage and lymphocyte activity, increasing susceptibility to opportunistic pathogens such as *Aeromonas hydrophila* and *Vibrio spp.*. Additionally, oxygen deficiency promotes anaerobic bacterial growth in sediments, leading to the production of toxic gases like hydrogen sulfide and methane. Thus, DO management is a key preventive measure in fish health management programs.

The **pH** of water measures its acidity or alkalinity, defined as the negative logarithm of hydrogen ion concentration. It profoundly influences fish physiology, water chemistry, and the bioavailability of nutrients and toxins.

Most freshwater and marine fish species thrive in a **pH range between 6.5 and 8.5**. Extreme deviations can cause physiological stress, gill irritation, and mortality. Acidic water ($pH < 6$) increases the solubility of toxic metals like aluminum and iron, which damage gill tissues and impair respiration. On the other hand, highly alkaline water ($pH > 9$) can disrupt ion regulation and cause ammonia toxicity.The gills are particularly sensitive to pH fluctuations. Acidic conditions damage gill epithelium, impairing gas exchange and ion regulation. Changes in pH also alter the blood acid-base balance, affecting oxygen transport and metabolic functions. In addition, extreme pH levels interfere with enzyme activity, nutrient absorption, and reproductive success.

pH interacts strongly with other parameters, particularly ammonia. As pH increases, the proportion of toxic un-ionized ammonia (NH_3) rises, significantly increasing toxicity. Similarly, low pH enhances the solubility of heavy metals, aggravating their harmful effects. Therefore, pH stability is crucial for maintaining both chemical and biological equilibrium in aquaculture systems.Regular monitoring and buffering are essential to maintain stable pH. In pond systems, **liming** with calcium carbonate or dolomite is a common practice to increase alkalinity and stabilize pH. In recirculating systems, biological filtration and the use of buffering agents help counteract acidification from nitrification processes. Sudden pH fluctuations should be avoided, as they cause acute stress and increase disease vulnerability.

Temperature is one of the most influential environmental factors governing fish metabolism, growth, immune response, and reproduction. Being **poikilothermic (cold-blooded)** animals, fish cannot regulate their body temperature internally; thus, their physiological processes directly depend on the ambient water temperature.Metabolic reactions in fish are temperature-dependent. Within an optimal thermal range, increased temperature enhances enzymatic activity, digestion, and growth rates. However, beyond the upper threshold, metabolic demand exceeds oxygen supply, leading to stress and mortality. Similarly, at low temperatures, metabolism slows, suppressing feeding and immune activity.Each species has a distinct **thermal optimum** and tolerance range. For example, **coldwater species** like trout prefer 12–18°C, **warmwater species** such as tilapia thrive between 25–30°C, and **tropical species** like catfish can tolerate slightly higher temperatures. Deviations outside these ranges, even for short durations, can impair performance and health.Temperature fluctuations influence pathogen virulence and host immunity. Many bacterial and parasitic diseases, such as **Columnaris disease** and **Ichthyophthiriasis (white spot disease)**, are temperature-dependent. Warm conditions often accelerate pathogen multiplication and disease progression, while rapid temperature drops can cause stress-induced immunosuppression. Stable thermal conditions are, therefore, vital for disease prevention.

In open pond systems, shading, aeration, and water exchange help mitigate temperature extremes. In recirculating aquaculture systems (RAS), heaters and chillers allow precise control, maintaining optimal thermal conditions year-round. Selecting species suited to local climatic conditions is a sustainable approach to minimize thermal stress.Ammonia is a **major nitrogenous waste product** resulting from protein metabolism and excretion through gills and urine. It exists in two forms in water: **un-ionized ammonia (NH_3)**, which is highly toxic, and **ionized ammonium (NH_4^+)**, which is comparatively harmless. The proportion of these two forms depends on pH and temperature — higher pH and temperature favor the more toxic un-ionized form.

Ammonia accumulation results primarily from the breakdown of uneaten feed, fish excreta, and microbial decomposition of organic matter. Overfeeding, poor water exchange, and inadequate biofiltration in intensive systems often lead to elevated ammonia concentrations.Even low concentrations of un-ionized ammonia (0.02–0.05 mg/L) can cause chronic stress and gill damage. Ammonia interferes with oxygen transport by increasing blood pH and reducing hemoglobin affinity for oxygen. High levels cause gill hyperplasia, mucus secretion, lethargy, and reduced feeding. Prolonged exposure leads to impaired growth, reduced immunity, and increased susceptibility to pathogens. At concentrations above 1 mg/L NH_3, mortality is common.Maintaining low ammonia levels requires effective biofiltration, aeration, and water exchange. **Nitrifying bacteria** in biological filters convert ammonia to nitrite and then to nitrate, a less toxic compound. Regular removal of organic waste, controlled feeding, and maintaining appropriate pH (below 8.5) and temperature (below 30°C) minimize the accumulation of toxic ammonia. The use of **zeolite** and other ammonia-binding agents also provides temporary relief in emergency situations.

Water quality parameters are not isolated factors; they are **interconnected** and influence each other. For instance, temperature affects oxygen solubility and metabolic oxygen demand; pH influences ammonia toxicity; and DO affects nitrification rates. A change in one parameter can cascade through the system, disturbing the entire ecological balance. Therefore, water quality management in aquaculture must adopt an integrated approach that monitors and maintains equilibrium among all essential parameters simultaneously.The parameters of dissolved oxygen, pH, temperature, and ammonia collectively define the environmental quality in aquaculture systems. These factors directly affect the physiological processes, immune status, and overall health of cultured fish. Imbalances lead to stress, reduced growth, and increased disease outbreaks, undermining productivity and sustainability. Regular water quality monitoring, coupled with good management practices—such as aeration, filtration, feeding control, and pH buffering—is vital for maintaining stable and healthy aquatic environments. As aquaculture continues to intensify, technological advancements such as real-time water quality sensors, automated aeration, and biofiltration systems will play an increasingly important role in safeguarding fish welfare and ensuring optimal production efficiency.

4.2 STOCKING DENSITY, FEEDING PRACTICES, AND HANDLING STRESS

The success of aquaculture operations depends not only on water quality and nutrition but also on optimal management of **stocking density, feeding practices, and handling procedures**, all of which directly influence fish health, welfare, and disease resistance. These three factors are closely interlinked and determine the overall physiological stability of cultured fish. Poor management in any of these areas induces stress, compromises immune function, and increases susceptibility to opportunistic pathogens. Understanding how these husbandry parameters affect fish physiology and behavior is therefore fundamental to sustainable aquaculture production.

Stocking density refers to the number or biomass of fish per unit volume or surface area of water. It is a critical management variable that affects growth performance, water quality, feed utilization, and social interactions among fish. While high stocking densities are often used to maximize production per unit area, overcrowding can lead to detrimental effects on fish health and welfare.

At high densities, fish experience chronic stress due to competition for space, oxygen, and food. This triggers the **hypothalamic-pituitary-interrenal (HPI) axis**, leading to elevated cortisol levels, which in turn suppress immunity and alter metabolic processes. Prolonged exposure to stress hormones reduces appetite, growth rates, and reproductive performance. Furthermore, crowding alters social behavior—dominant individuals may monopolize feed, while subordinate fish become malnourished and immunocompromised. Aggression, fin damage, and abnormal swimming patterns are common signs of overstocking stress.Overcrowded systems produce large amounts of metabolic waste, leading to rapid accumulation of ammonia, nitrite, and carbon dioxide. As oxygen demand increases, dissolved oxygen levels decline, creating hypoxic conditions that favor pathogenic microbial proliferation. Diseases such as **columnaris (Flavobacterium columnare), bacterial gill disease**, and **fin rot** are frequently associated with high stocking densities. These conditions not only facilitate pathogen transmission but also weaken fish defenses due to increased mucus damage and reduced energy reserves.The ideal stocking density varies with species, size, system type, and management practices. For instance, Nile tilapia may tolerate up to 60–80 kg/m^3 in recirculating systems with efficient aeration, while carp and catfish require lower densities in pond environments. In general, stocking should aim for a balance between productivity and welfare, maintaining water quality and minimizing chronic stress. Frequent monitoring of behavior, feed intake, and water parameters provides valuable indicators for density adjustment.Proper system design, adequate water circulation, and regular size grading help reduce stress associated with crowding. In addition, **all-in-all-out culture systems**, where fish are stocked and harvested simultaneously, minimize disease transmission between age groups.

Implementing biosecurity protocols and quarantine procedures before stocking also reduces the introduction of pathogens into high-density environments.

Feeding management is another cornerstone of healthy aquaculture. The **type, quality, frequency, and method of feeding** directly influence growth performance, water quality, and disease resistance. Nutritional imbalances or feeding errors often lead to physiological stress, metabolic disorders, and increased pathogen susceptibility.A well-balanced diet ensures adequate protein, lipids, carbohydrates, vitamins, and minerals to support growth, reproduction, and immune function. Deficiencies in essential nutrients—such as vitamin C, E, selenium, or omega-3 fatty acids—impair antioxidant defense mechanisms, making fish more prone to oxidative stress and infections. For example, vitamin C deficiency weakens collagen synthesis, leading to deformities and hemorrhagic symptoms, while vitamin E deficiency causes muscular dystrophy and poor immunity.

Excessive feeding not only wastes expensive feed but also deteriorates water quality. Uneaten feed decomposes, increasing ammonia and nitrite concentrations and depleting dissolved oxygen. The resulting poor water quality induces chronic stress and enhances the virulence of pathogens such as *Aeromonas*, *Edwardsiella*, and *Vibrio* species. Overfeeding also predisposes fish to fatty liver disease, obesity, and reproductive problems.In contrast, underfeeding results in nutrient deficiencies, reduced energy availability, and stunted growth. Malnourished fish exhibit poor coloration, weak immune responses, and delayed wound healing. Chronic undernutrition suppresses lymphocyte proliferation and antibody production, rendering fish highly vulnerable to bacterial and parasitic infections.The frequency and timing of feeding should correspond to the species' natural feeding habits, temperature, and activity patterns. Carnivorous fish require multiple small feedings per day, while omnivorous and herbivorous species can adapt to fewer meals. Automated feeders and demand-feeding systems help maintain consistency and prevent feed competition. Observing feeding behavior is an effective tool for assessing fish health—lethargic or disoriented feeding responses often indicate stress or disease onset.In recent years, functional feeds containing probiotics, prebiotics, immunostimulants, and herbal extracts have gained attention for enhancing disease resistance and gut health. Additives like β-glucans, garlic extract, and *Bacillus* probiotics improve intestinal microflora balance and boost innate immunity.

These dietary interventions reduce the need for antibiotics and enhance resilience against environmental stressors.

Handling is an unavoidable part of aquaculture operations, necessary for grading, vaccination, sampling, or transportation. However, **improper handling practices** can cause severe physiological stress, physical injury, and increased mortality. Fish are extremely sensitive to mechanical disturbances, and even short-term handling can trigger a cascade of stress responses.When fish are handled, captured, or netted, they undergo an immediate primary stress response characterized by elevated cortisol, glucose, and lactate levels. Secondary responses include altered osmoregulation, reduced immunity, and increased susceptibility to opportunistic infections. The tertiary phase manifests as behavioral changes such as loss of equilibrium, erratic swimming, and suppressed feeding. If stress persists, chronic conditions like gill damage, mucosal erosion, and fin necrosis can develop.

Handling can damage the protective mucus layer, scales, and fins, creating entry points for pathogens. Rough nets, dry hands, and inappropriate equipment exacerbate physical injuries. Wound sites become colonized by bacteria like *Aeromonas hydrophila* and *Pseudomonas fluorescens*, leading to ulcerative conditions. Therefore, minimizing mechanical damage is a critical aspect of fish health management.Handling should be conducted as gently and infrequently as possible. Nets with soft, knotless mesh should be used, and fish should remain submerged during transfer to minimize air exposure. The use of anesthetics such as **tricaine methanesulfonate (MS-222)** or **clove oil** can reduce stress during invasive procedures. Grading and sampling should be scheduled during cooler parts of the day to avoid thermal stress. After handling, fish should be allowed to recover in well-aerated, clean water with optimal temperature and oxygen conditions.Transportation is another major stressor involving confinement, crowding, and fluctuating environmental conditions. Oxygen depletion, ammonia accumulation, and temperature variations during transport can quickly lead to physiological exhaustion. To minimize these effects, water should be pre-oxygenated, and transport densities kept within safe limits. The addition of salt or stress-relieving agents like sodium chloride (2–5 ppt) helps maintain osmotic balance. Upon arrival, gradual acclimatization to temperature and water chemistry prevents shock and mortality.

Stocking density, feeding, and handling are interdependent components of aquaculture management. High stocking densities often increase competition for feed and oxygen, amplifying the effects of poor feeding practices. Overcrowding also necessitates frequent handling for grading and disease management, further compounding stress. Chronic exposure to multiple stressors results in a cumulative physiological burden, weakening fish immune defenses and facilitating disease outbreaks. Integrated management that balances these parameters is essential to maintain homeostasis and minimize risk.Stress acts as a silent precursor to most disease outbreaks in aquaculture. The release of cortisol under chronic stress conditions suppresses immune function, reduces antibody production, and alters mucosal defenses. Opportunistic pathogens that are normally harmless in healthy fish can become virulent under stress. For example, *Vibrio anguillarum*, *Aeromonas salmonicida*, and *Saprolegnia spp.* commonly exploit stressed hosts. Therefore, maintaining optimal husbandry conditions is not only a matter of welfare but also a primary line of disease prevention.Effective aquaculture management requires careful attention to stocking density, feeding practices, and handling procedures—three interrelated factors that determine the physiological well-being of fish. Overcrowding, improper feeding, and rough handling are major contributors to chronic stress, leading to suppressed immunity, poor growth, and disease outbreaks. Sustainable aquaculture practices should therefore emphasize balanced stocking rates, nutritionally adequate diets, gentle handling techniques, and minimal disturbance. Incorporating welfare-oriented management not only improves survival and productivity but also enhances product quality and consumer trust. Ultimately, the success of modern aquaculture depends on maintaining harmony between production efficiency and the biological needs of the cultured species.

4.3 BIOSECURITY AND HYGIENE IN AQUACULTURE FACILITIES

Biosecurity and hygiene are fundamental pillars of modern aquaculture management, essential for preventing the introduction, establishment, and spread of infectious diseases within and between aquatic animal populations. As aquaculture systems intensify and global trade in live aquatic organisms expands, the risk of disease outbreaks and transboundary pathogen transmission increases significantly. Effective biosecurity practices ensure not only the health and welfare of cultured species but also the sustainability and profitability of the entire aquaculture sector. Biosecurity encompasses a comprehensive set of preventive and control measures aimed at minimizing biological risks, while hygiene focuses on maintaining cleanliness and reducing microbial load within facilities. Together, these practices form the cornerstone of aquatic animal health management.

Biosecurity in aquaculture refers to a strategic and integrated approach designed to prevent the introduction and dissemination of infectious agents. It operates on the principle of "prevention is better than cure," recognizing that the economic and ecological cost of an outbreak far exceeds the investment in preventive measures. Biosecurity is not limited to disease control but also supports food safety, environmental protection, and sustainable resource use.

In aquaculture, biosecurity measures aim to:

- Prevent the **entry of pathogens** into farms (external biosecurity).
- Control the **spread of pathogens** within the farm (internal biosecurity).
- Limit the **release of pathogens** into the surrounding environment (environmental biosecurity).

Failure in any of these components can result in catastrophic disease events. For instance, outbreaks of **White Spot Syndrome Virus (WSSV)** in shrimp or **Infectious Salmon Anemia (ISA)** in salmon farms have demonstrated the devastating impact of inadequate biosecurity on global aquaculture production and trade.

2. Sources and Pathways of Disease Introduction

Pathogens can enter aquaculture systems through multiple routes, often linked to lapses in management practices. Common sources include:

- **Infected seed stock or broodstock** introduced without proper health screening.
- **Contaminated water sources** carrying pathogens from other farms or wild populations.
- **Vectors and carriers**, such as birds, crustaceans, mollusks, or aquatic insects, that transfer pathogens mechanically or biologically.
- **Human activities**, including workers, visitors, or equipment moving between farms.
- **Feed and organic materials**, especially when using raw or unprocessed animal products.

- **Environmental factors**, such as runoff water, flooding, or poor drainage connecting infected and healthy farms.

Recognizing these pathways is the first step in designing effective biosecurity protocols that block or mitigate potential transmission routes.

3. Components of an Effective Biosecurity Program

A comprehensive biosecurity program integrates several key components tailored to the specific facility type, species, and culture system. These include **quarantine, health screening, facility design, movement control, disinfection, and record-keeping**.All new broodstock, fry, or fingerlings must undergo quarantine before introduction into production units. A **minimum quarantine period of 2–4 weeks** allows observation for clinical signs of disease and laboratory testing for pathogens. Health certification from recognized laboratories ensures the use of pathogen-free stock. This measure is critical in preventing the introduction of transboundary diseases like Koi Herpesvirus (KHV) or Epizootic Ulcerative Syndrome (EUS).Biosecure facility design plays a major role in disease prevention. Separate units for hatchery, nursery, and grow-out stages reduce cross-contamination risks. Water supply systems should be equipped with **filtration, sedimentation, and disinfection units (e.g., UV sterilization or ozonation)** to eliminate pathogens. Flow patterns should prevent backflow from potentially contaminated ponds. Adequate drainage and waste treatment systems minimize environmental pollution and pathogen accumulation.Restricting movement of people, vehicles, and equipment between units or farms is vital. Entry points should be equipped with **footbaths, hand sanitizers, and vehicle disinfection stations**. Visitors and staff must follow hygiene protocols, wear protective clothing, and avoid contact with multiple facilities in a short period. Equipment such as nets, buckets, and aerators should be assigned to specific tanks or disinfected thoroughly between uses.Common disinfectants include **chlorine compounds, potassium permanganate, iodine solutions, and formalin**, applied at recommended concentrations. After harvesting or disease outbreaks, ponds should be **drained, dried, and limed** to eliminate residual pathogens. Feed storage areas and water pipes should also be cleaned periodically to prevent biofilm formation and microbial growth.

Accurate documentation of stocking, feeding, treatments, mortalities, and water quality is essential for early disease detection and traceability. Health surveillance programs involving **routine sampling, microscopic examinations, and molecular diagnostics** enable timely intervention before widespread outbreaks occur. A culture of continuous monitoring and record review enhances preparedness and accountability.Hygiene refers to maintaining a clean and sanitary environment to reduce the risk of infection. While biosecurity deals with strategic prevention, hygiene focuses on daily operational cleanliness and personal practices.Workers play a crucial role in pathogen transmission. Proper hygiene protocols—such as handwashing, wearing clean protective clothing, and using footbaths—must be strictly enforced. Employees should avoid handling fish if they have open wounds and must sanitize themselves before and after working in culture areas. Training programs should emphasize the importance of hygiene as part of farm culture rather than as a periodic requirement.All areas of the farm, including storage rooms, feed areas, and laboratories, should be maintained in a clean state. Organic waste such as uneaten feed, dead fish, and sludge should be removed promptly. **Dead or diseased fish** must be disposed of safely by **burial, incineration, or rendering**, rather than discarded in nearby water bodies. Sludge and sediment should be treated or composted to prevent nutrient buildup and anaerobic conditions that harbor pathogens.Feed should be stored in dry, rodent-free areas to prevent contamination and fungal growth. Using **heat-treated or pelleted feeds** minimizes pathogen introduction compared to raw feeds. Feeding equipment and water testing tools should be disinfected daily and not shared between tanks or ponds. Aerators, pipes, and filters must be regularly cleaned to prevent biofilm-associated bacterial colonization.Biosecurity requirements vary across production stages. In **hatcheries**, maintaining pathogen-free broodstock and disinfecting eggs are essential. **Egg disinfection** with iodophor or hydrogen peroxide before incubation prevents the spread of fungal and bacterial infections. Hatchery water should be filtered and UV-treated to maintain sterility.Separate equipment should be used for each pond, and water should never be recirculated from one pond to another without treatment. Stocking density should be optimized to reduce stress and disease transmission. Regular health monitoring, including observation of feeding behavior and swimming activity, aids early detection of problems.

Biosecurity extends beyond farm boundaries to include the surrounding environment. Effluents from aquaculture facilities can contain pathogens, organic waste, and chemicals that contaminate natural water bodies. Implementing **effluent treatment systems**—including sedimentation ponds, biofilters, and constructed wetlands—reduces microbial load and nutrient discharge. Farms should avoid sharing common water sources or drainage channels with neighboring facilities to minimize disease spread.Proper waste management is equally critical. Sludge, mortalities, and feed waste must be disposed of following environmental regulations. Composting, biogas generation, or rendering are sustainable options that convert waste into useful products while maintaining hygiene.Even with stringent biosecurity, disease outbreaks may occur. Therefore, farms should have a **contingency plan** outlining procedures for disease diagnosis, isolation, treatment, and communication with authorities. Quarantining affected units, restricting movement, and disinfection of surrounding areas are immediate priorities. Coordination with national aquatic animal health services ensures timely reporting and containment of emerging diseases. Staff training in emergency biosecurity response enhances preparedness and reduces the spread of infection.

Effective biosecurity practices yield significant economic benefits by reducing disease-related losses and improving production efficiency. Although implementation requires initial investment in infrastructure and training, the long-term savings from avoided outbreaks far outweigh the costs. Governments and international bodies, such as the **World Organisation for Animal Health (WOAH)** and the **Food and Agriculture Organization (FAO)**, have established guidelines and certification schemes for biosecure aquaculture. Compliance with these standards also facilitates access to export markets by ensuring the production of pathogen-free and safe aquatic products.Modern aquaculture increasingly incorporates **digital biosecurity systems** using sensors, automated feeders, and remote monitoring to detect anomalies in water quality and fish behavior. Technologies like **blockchain traceability** enhance transparency in supply chains, while **machine learning models** predict disease risks based on environmental data. The integration of such innovations strengthens preventive biosecurity and supports evidence-based management decisions.Biosecurity and hygiene are indispensable elements of responsible aquaculture. They represent proactive defense mechanisms against infectious diseases, ensuring the sustainability, profitability, and environmental compatibility of fish farming operations. A robust biosecurity framework—encompassing quarantine, disinfection, movement control, and environmental management—forms the first line of defense against pathogen introduction and spread.

CHAPTER 5

DIAGNOSTIC METHODS IN FISH PATHOLOGY

5.1 Diagnosis of Fish Diseases: Clinical, Laboratory, and Molecular Approaches

Effective disease diagnosis in aquaculture is essential for maintaining fish health, minimizing economic losses, and ensuring sustainable production. Early and accurate diagnosis enables timely intervention, preventing the spread of infectious agents and improving treatment outcomes. The diagnostic process in aquaculture is multifaceted, encompassing **clinical observations, behavioral assessments, laboratory analyses, and advanced molecular and immunological techniques.** Each level of diagnosis provides complementary information, contributing to a holistic understanding of fish health status and the underlying causes of disease.

1. Clinical Observation and Behavioral Symptoms

Clinical observation forms the **first line of disease detection** in aquaculture. Experienced farmers and fish health professionals can often recognize early signs of illness by observing changes in fish behavior, appearance, and performance. These visible or behavioral abnormalities are often the initial indicators of physiological distress caused by pathogens, poor water quality, nutritional imbalance, or environmental stress.

Behavioral Symptoms:

Behavioral changes are among the most reliable early signs of disease. Healthy fish exhibit active swimming, balanced buoyancy, coordinated movement, and prompt feeding responses. In contrast, diseased or stressed fish often display lethargy, erratic swimming, loss of equilibrium, reduced feeding, and isolation from the group. Common behavioral symptoms include:

- **Abnormal swimming patterns:** Fish may swim in circles, hang near the surface, or lie at the bottom.
- **Loss of appetite:** A marked decrease in feed intake often precedes clinical disease.
- **Gasping at the water surface:** Indicative of low dissolved oxygen or gill infections caused by parasites, bacteria, or fungi.

- **Rubbing or flashing behavior:** Fish may rub against tank walls or substrates due to irritation from ectoparasites or skin infections.
- **Crowding near inlets or aerators:** Suggests oxygen depletion, toxic compounds, or gill damage.

Continuous observation of these behaviors allows early identification of problems before mortality occurs.

Clinical Signs:

Clinical examination involves assessing the external and internal appearance of fish for abnormalities. Common **external signs** include discoloration, fin rot, exophthalmia (pop-eye), skin ulcers, hemorrhages, scale loss, and excessive mucus production. Lesions may appear as localized ulcers, necrosis, or cotton-like fungal growths. The **gills** may appear pale, swollen, or covered with mucus, indicating parasitic or bacterial infections. The **abdomen** may appear distended due to ascites or organ enlargement. Internally, necrosis or congestion in organs such as the liver, kidney, or spleen may be evident during necropsy.

c. Importance of Record Keeping:

Accurate recording of behavioral and clinical symptoms, mortality patterns, environmental parameters, and recent management changes provides essential clues for diagnosis. Such records facilitate correlation between environmental fluctuations and disease outbreaks, supporting differential diagnosis and effective treatment planning.

2. Laboratory Diagnosis: Microscopy, Culture, and Histopathology

While clinical observations provide preliminary evidence, **laboratory diagnosis** confirms the causative agent and helps determine appropriate control measures. Laboratory methods range from simple microscopic examinations to complex culture and histological analyses.

Microscopic Examination:

Microscopy is a rapid, cost-effective, and widely used diagnostic tool in aquaculture. It allows visualization of **parasites, bacteria, fungi, and cellular changes** directly from fish tissues or smears.

- **Wet mount preparations** of skin, gill, and fin samples are examined under light microscopy to detect ectoparasites such as *Ichthyophthirius multifiliis*, *Trichodina*, *Gyrodactylus*, and *Dactylogyrus*.
- **Gram staining** helps distinguish between Gram-positive and Gram-negative bacteria, aiding preliminary bacterial identification.
- **Blood smears** can reveal hemoparasites or changes in leukocyte morphology associated with systemic infections.
- **Fungal elements** (hyphae or spores) can be visualized in tissue imprints stained with lactophenol cotton blue or Giemsa stains.

Microscopy is indispensable for quick field diagnosis, allowing farmers to initiate treatment while awaiting confirmatory results.

b. Microbial Culture:

Culture methods are the gold standard for identifying bacterial and fungal pathogens. Samples from infected organs (kidney, spleen, gill, or lesion tissue) are inoculated onto selective media under aseptic conditions.

- Common media include **Tryptic Soy Agar (TSA), Brain Heart Infusion Agar (BHIA), and Nutrient Agar** for general bacterial growth.
- **Thiosulfate-Citrate-Bile Salts-Sucrose (TCBS)** agar is used for *Vibrio* species, while **Edwardsiella** and **Aeromonas** species are isolated using specific enrichment media.
- Fungi such as *Saprolegnia* are cultured on **Sabouraud Dextrose Agar (SDA)**.

Colonies are examined for morphology, pigmentation, hemolysis, and biochemical characteristics using tests like **oxidase, catalase, and sugar fermentation**. These phenotypic profiles help identify pathogens at the species level. Although culture methods are time-consuming, they remain crucial for antibiotic sensitivity testing, guiding effective therapeutic management.

c. Histopathology:

Histopathological examination provides detailed insights into tissue-level changes and disease mechanisms. Tissues (gills, liver, kidney, spleen, and intestine) are fixed in **10% neutral buffered formalin**, sectioned, stained (commonly with hematoxylin and eosin), and examined under a microscope.

- Lesions such as necrosis, inflammation, cellular infiltration, or granuloma formation can indicate specific infections.
- For instance, **melanomacrophage centers** suggest chronic inflammation, while **vacuolation** may indicate viral infections like lymphocystis.
- Special stains such as **Periodic Acid-Schiff (PAS)** or **Ziehl-Neelsen** may be used for fungal or acid-fast bacterial identification.

Histopathology not only aids in confirming diagnosis but also helps assess disease progression, severity, and organ involvement.

3. Molecular and Immunological Diagnostic Tools

Advancements in molecular biology and immunology have revolutionized aquatic disease diagnosis, providing **rapid, sensitive, and specific** detection of pathogens, even before clinical signs appear. These modern techniques complement traditional methods and are now standard tools in disease surveillance and certification programs.

Polymerase Chain Reaction (PCR):

PCR is a highly sensitive molecular technique used to detect pathogen DNA or RNA in fish tissues, water, or environmental samples. It amplifies specific genetic sequences unique to the target pathogen, allowing detection even when present in minute quantities. Variants such as **nested**

PCR, multiplex PCR, quantitative real-time PCR (qPCR), and reverse transcription PCR (RT-PCR) enhance sensitivity and specificity.

- PCR is widely used for detecting viral diseases like **Koi Herpesvirus (KHV), Infectious Pancreatic Necrosis Virus (IPNV), and White Spot Syndrome Virus (WSSV)** in shrimp.
- qPCR provides quantitative data, enabling estimation of pathogen load and monitoring of infection dynamics.

PCR's major advantages include rapid results, high specificity, and applicability in asymptomatic carrier detection. However, it requires specialized equipment and trained personnel.

b. Enzyme-Linked Immunosorbent Assay (ELISA):

ELISA is an immunological test that detects specific **antigens or antibodies** in fish serum or tissue extracts using enzyme-labeled antibodies. It is widely used in surveillance programs for viral and bacterial diseases such as **Infectious Salmon Anemia (ISA)** and **Viral Hemorrhagic Septicemia (VHS)**.
There are several ELISA formats, including **direct, indirect, and sandwich ELISA**, depending on whether the antigen or antibody is being detected.

- The presence of **specific antibodies** indicates prior exposure or infection, while **antigen detection** confirms active infection. ELISA is valued for its ability to process large sample numbers with high accuracy and minimal labor.

c. Immunofluorescence and Immunohistochemistry (IHC):

These techniques use fluorescent or enzyme-labeled antibodies to visualize pathogens within tissues.

- **Direct immunofluorescence (DIF)** detects antigen presence in tissue sections or smears.

- **IHC** combines histology with antibody labeling, allowing visualization of the exact tissue location of pathogens. These tools provide insight into pathogen distribution and host tissue interaction.

d. Other Molecular Techniques:

Advanced molecular approaches such as **Loop-Mediated Isothermal Amplification (LAMP), DNA hybridization**, and **Next-Generation Sequencing (NGS)** are gaining importance.

- **LAMP** offers a rapid, field-deployable alternative to PCR, requiring minimal equipment.
- **NGS** enables whole-genome sequencing of pathogens, discovery of novel agents, and analysis of microbial communities in aquaculture environments. Such high-throughput tools are pivotal for epidemiological studies and early warning systems.

4. Integration of Diagnostic Approaches

The most effective diagnosis relies on **a combination of clinical, laboratory, and molecular findings.** Field-level observation initiates suspicion, while laboratory tests confirm etiology. Molecular and immunological assays provide high specificity, allowing detection of latent infections or co-infections. Integration of these methods enhances diagnostic accuracy, speeds up decision-making, and improves biosecurity management in aquaculture operations.

The diagnosis of fish diseases in aquaculture requires a systematic and multidisciplinary approach. Beginning with **clinical observation and behavioral assessment**, progressing through **microscopic and cultural analyses**, and culminating in **molecular and immunological testing**, each diagnostic level adds precision and reliability. Traditional methods remain invaluable for their practicality and cost-effectiveness, while modern molecular tools enable rapid and specific pathogen detection essential for disease surveillance and certification. By integrating these diagnostic strategies, aquaculture practitioners can ensure early detection, effective treatment, and sustainable management of aquatic animal health — a cornerstone of global food security and environmental sustainability.

REFERENCES

[1] World Organisation for Animal Health (WOAH) guidelines on disease reporting and biosecurity.

[2] Food and Agriculture Organization (FAO) guidelines on aquaculture and disease management.

[3] Pat Mooney's work on biopiracy.

[4] National Policy for the Empowerment of Women, 2001.

[5] TRYSEM: Training of Rural Youth For Self Employment was launched on 15th August 1979 which is still continuing.

[6] IDBI: Industrial Development Bank of India (IDBI) set up the Mahila Udyan Nidhi (MUN) and Mahila Vikas Nidhi (MVN) schemes to help women entrepreneurs.

[7] SIDBI: Small Industries Development Bank of India (SIDBI) has special schemes for financial assistance to women entrepreneurs.

[8] National Alliance of Young Entrepreneurs (NAYE) assists the women entrepreneurs in getting better access to capital, infrastructure and markets.

TABLE OF CONTENTS

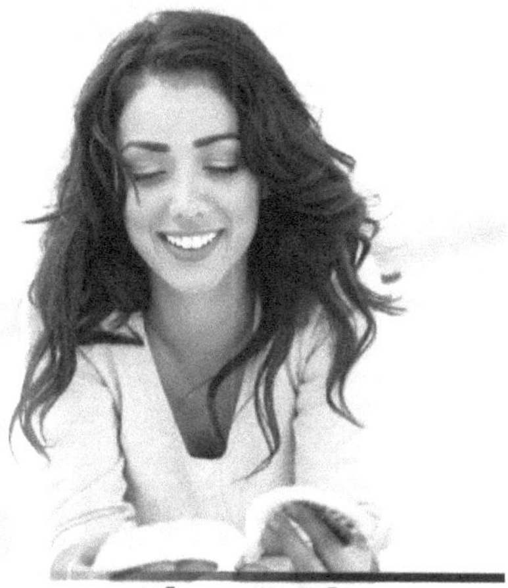

Kolibri 360 GmbH
Ferdinand-Jühlke-Straße 7
99095 Erfurt, Deutschland
produktsicherheit@kolibri360.de

Druck:
CPI Druckdienstleistungen GmbH
im Auftrag der
Kolibri 360 GmbH
Ferdinand-Jühlke-Str. 7
99095 Erfurt